The Peptic Ulcer Solution

Cutting-Edge Therapies and Best Practices

Table of Contents:

"The Peptic Ulcer Solution: Cutting-Edge Therapies and Best Practices"

Introduction

"The Peptic Ulcer Solution: Cutting-Edge Therapies and Best Practices"

Welcome to "The Peptic Ulcer Solution: Cutting-Edge Therapies and Best Practices." This comprehensive guide is designed to be your definitive resource for understanding, managing, and overcoming the challenges of peptic ulcers. Whether you are a patient seeking relief from the distressing symptoms of this condition or a healthcare professional looking to enhance your knowledge and treatment strategies, this book aims to equip you with the latest insights and evidence-based approaches in peptic ulcer management.

Peptic ulcers, affecting millions of individuals worldwide, remain a prevalent gastrointestinal issue with potentially serious consequences if left untreated. These sores, found in the lining of the stomach, upper small intestine, or esophagus, can lead to discomfort, pain, and complications that interfere with daily life. In recent years, advancements in medical science and innovative therapies have revolutionized the way we approach peptic ulcers, offering new hope and opportunities for healing.

Our journey through this book begins with a comprehensive exploration of the fundamentals, shedding light on the nature of peptic ulcers, their distinct types, and the underlying causes and risk factors. Understanding the symptoms and potential complications is crucial for early detection and effective management. Through this knowledge, patients and healthcare providers can collaborate in making informed decisions for personalized treatment plans.

Chapter by chapter, we delve into the diagnostic methods utilized to accurately identify peptic ulcers and their causes. From endoscopic procedures to cutting-edge imaging technologies and laboratory studies, we navigate the various tools available for precise assessment. Furthermore, the crucial role of detecting and addressing Helicobacter pylori infection, a common trigger for peptic ulcers, is extensively explored.

Throughout this book, we provide a comprehensive overview of traditional treatments, including acid-suppressing medications like antacids, H2 blockers, and proton pump inhibitors (PPIs). Understanding the mechanisms and limitations of these therapies is vital for patients and clinicians alike. However, we go beyond conventional approaches, examining the latest advancements in peptic ulcer treatments. From mucosal protective agents and combination therapies to the use of probiotics, we explore the cutting-edge options transforming the landscape of ulcer care.

Recognizing that peptic ulcer management extends beyond medical interventions, we also investigate the crucial role of lifestyle modifications. Diet, stress management, smoking, and alcohol consumption all play pivotal roles in ulcer development and healing. By empowering individuals to make informed choices, we aim to enhance treatment outcomes and reduce the risk of recurrence.

In pursuit of holistic healing, this book embraces integrative approaches to peptic ulcer care. Herbal remedies, natural supplements, and complementary therapies like acupuncture and meditation are investigated, providing readers with a comprehensive understanding of the potential benefits and risks associated with these practices.

For those facing complicated peptic ulcers or requiring surgical intervention, we present a thorough analysis of surgical options, indications, and postoperative care. Additionally, we emphasize the importance of long-term follow-up and proactive strategies for preventing ulcer recurrence.

Peptic ulcers can affect people of all ages and backgrounds, and we address specific considerations for managing ulcers in special populations such as children, pregnant individuals, the elderly, and immunocompromised patients.

Finally, as we glimpse into the future of peptic ulcer management, we explore the promising therapies on the horizon, the concept of personalized medicine, and the collaborative efforts driving progress in this field. The book culminates with empowering stories of individuals who have successfully managed their peptic ulcers and, in doing so, offer hope and inspiration to all readers on their journey towards healing.

Our aim with "The Peptic Ulcer Solution: Cutting-Edge Therapies and Best Practices" is to provide a comprehensive, authoritative, and accessible resource that will empower readers with the knowledge and tools they need to effectively manage peptic ulcers. It is our sincere hope that this book serves as a beacon of hope, guiding patients and healthcare providers towards a future free from the burden of peptic ulceration. Let us embark on this journey together, empowering ourselves and others to face the challenges of peptic ulcers with confidence and determination.

Chapter 1

Understanding Peptic Ulcers

Peptic ulcers are a common gastrointestinal disorder that affects millions of individuals worldwide. In this chapter, we will delve into the fundamental aspects of peptic ulcers, shedding light on their nature, classification, causes, risk factors, and the importance of recognizing symptoms and complications.

What are Peptic Ulcers?

Peptic ulcers are painful sores that develop on the inner lining of the stomach, upper small intestine (duodenum), or esophagus. These ulcers form when the protective mucous layer that shields the digestive tract from stomach acid and digestive enzymes is compromised, leading to erosions in the lining. The erosion exposes the sensitive tissues to the corrosive substances, causing inflammation and the characteristic burning pain associated with peptic ulcers.

Types of Peptic Ulcers: Gastric vs. Duodenal

Peptic ulcers are primarily categorized based on their location within the digestive system. Gastric ulcers occur in the stomach lining, while duodenal ulcers develop in the first part of the small intestine known as the duodenum. Although both types share similar symptoms and causes, their locations can influence the presentation and response to treatment.

Causes and Risk Factors

Understanding the underlying causes and risk factors for peptic ulcers is crucial for effective management and prevention. The primary cause of most peptic ulcers is the presence of Helicobacter pylori (H. pylori) bacteria. H. pylori infects the lining of the stomach and duodenum, weakening the protective mucous barrier and making it susceptible to damage from stomach acid.

In addition to H. pylori infection, other risk factors include the long-term use of nonsteroidal anti-inflammatory drugs (NSAIDs) such as aspirin or ibuprofen, which can irritate the stomach lining. Smoking and excessive alcohol consumption are also associated with an increased risk of developing peptic ulcers. Furthermore, certain medical conditions, such as Zollinger-Ellison syndrome, a rare disorder that leads to excessive stomach acid production, can contribute to peptic ulcer formation.

Recognizing Symptoms and Complications

Peptic ulcers can cause a range of symptoms, and their severity can vary from person to person. Common symptoms include a burning or gnawing pain in the upper abdomen, often occurring between meals and in the early hours of the morning. The pain can be temporarily relieved by consuming food or antacids. Other symptoms may include bloating, belching, nausea, and in some cases, vomiting.

Failure to diagnose and treat peptic ulcers promptly can lead to potentially serious complications. These complications may include bleeding ulcers, which can result in blood in the stool or vomit, and perforated ulcers, where the ulcer creates a hole in the stomach or intestinal wall, causing severe abdominal pain and requiring immediate medical attention.

In this chapter, we have laid the foundation for a comprehensive understanding of peptic ulcers. By recognizing the different types of ulcers, understanding their causes and risk factors, and being aware of the symptoms and potential complications, individuals can be better equipped to seek timely medical attention and embark on the journey towards effective peptic ulcer management. In the following chapters, we will explore the diagnostic tools, treatment options, lifestyle modifications, and promising advancements that form the basis of "The Peptic Ulcer Solution: Cutting-Edge Therapies and Best Practices."

Chapter 2

Diagnosing Peptic Ulcers

Timely and accurate diagnosis is paramount in effectively managing peptic ulcers. In this chapter, we will explore the essential steps involved in diagnosing peptic ulcers, highlighting the significance of early detection and the various diagnostic methods available to healthcare professionals.

The Importance of Early Detection

Early detection of peptic ulcers is crucial to prevent potential complications and ensure appropriate treatment. Left untreated, peptic ulcers can lead to bleeding, perforation, or even stomach obstruction. Therefore, recognizing the symptoms and seeking medical attention promptly can significantly impact the outcome of peptic ulcer management. Early intervention not only aids in pain relief but also reduces the risk of further damage to the digestive tract.

Medical History and Physical Examination

The first step in diagnosing peptic ulcers involves a comprehensive medical history and physical examination. Healthcare professionals will inquire about the patient's symptoms, including the type and frequency of abdominal pain, associated gastrointestinal symptoms, and any factors that alleviate or worsen the pain. They will also inquire about the use of medications, particularly NSAIDs and aspirin, as well as the patient's alcohol consumption and smoking history, which are known risk factors for peptic ulcers.

During the physical examination, the healthcare provider will assess the patient's abdomen for tenderness, bloating, or any signs of discomfort. They will also check for evidence of gastrointestinal bleeding, such as pallor or signs of anemia.

Diagnostic Tests: Endoscopy, Imaging, and Laboratory Studies

To confirm the presence of peptic ulcers and identify their location, healthcare professionals may recommend various diagnostic tests.

Endoscopy: Upper gastrointestinal endoscopy is a common procedure used to visualize the inside of the esophagus, stomach, and duodenum. A thin, flexible tube with a tiny camera (endoscope) is inserted through the mouth and gently guided down the throat. This allows the healthcare provider to directly visualize any ulcers or inflammation in the gastrointestinal tract. During the procedure, if an ulcer is detected, the doctor may perform a biopsy to test for H. pylori infection or rule out other conditions.

Imaging Studies: In some cases, imaging tests such as X-rays, computed tomography (CT) scans, or magnetic resonance imaging (MRI) may be used to detect peptic ulcers or complications like perforation or obstruction.

Laboratory Studies: Blood tests can be conducted to assess the presence of H. pylori infection or to check for signs of anemia, which can occur due to chronic bleeding from an ulcer.

Identifying Helicobacter pylori Infection

As H. pylori infection is a significant cause of peptic ulcers, identifying its presence is crucial for effective management. This can be achieved through various methods, including:

Breath Test: The patient consumes a specific substance, and then their breath is analyzed for the presence of H. pylori-related compounds.

Stool Antigen Test: A stool sample is examined for H. pylori antigens, which are indicative of an active infection.

Biopsy: During endoscopy, a small tissue sample may be taken from the stomach lining for analysis to detect H. pylori.

Blood Test: Blood samples can be assessed for antibodies against H. pylori, indicating a past or current infection.

By utilizing these diagnostic methods, healthcare professionals can accurately diagnose peptic ulcers, assess their severity, and identify any underlying causes such as H. pylori infection. Armed with this information, a personalized treatment plan can be developed to effectively manage peptic ulcers and prevent potential complications. In the next chapters, we will delve into various treatment strategies, lifestyle modifications, and cutting-edge therapies that form the foundation of "The Peptic Ulcer Solution: Cutting-Edge Therapies and Best Practices."

Chapter 3
Traditional Treatments for Peptic Ulcers

Peptic ulcers have been managed effectively for decades using various traditional medications that aim to reduce stomach acid production and provide relief from symptoms. In this chapter, we will explore the different classes of acid-suppressing medications, their mechanisms of action, dosing guidelines, and potential side effects.

Acid-Suppressing Medications: Antacids, H2 Blockers, and Proton Pump Inhibitors (PPIs)

Acid-suppressing medications form the cornerstone of traditional peptic ulcer treatment. These drugs work by reducing the acidity of the stomach, thereby promoting ulcer healing and providing symptomatic relief.

- **Antacids:** Antacids are readily available over-the-counter and provide rapid relief from heartburn and indigestion. They work by neutralizing stomach acid, turning it into water and salt. Common antacid ingredients include aluminum hydroxide, magnesium hydroxide, calcium carbonate, and sodium bicarbonate.

- **H2 Blockers**: H2 blockers, also known as histamine H2-receptor antagonists, include medications such as ranitidine, famotidine, cimetidine, and nizatidine. They work by blocking histamine, a chemical that stimulates acid production, from binding to H2 receptors on the stomach cells. This leads to decreased acid secretion, reducing the irritation of the ulcerated mucosa.

- **Proton Pump Inhibitors (PPIs):** PPIs, such as omeprazole, lansoprazole, pantoprazole, rabeprazole, and esomeprazole, are among the most potent acid-suppressing medications. They work by irreversibly inhibiting the proton pump, a protein responsible for secreting acid into the stomach. PPIs provide long-lasting acid suppression, making them highly effective in promoting ulcer healing and preventing recurrence.

Understanding Antacids and Their Role in Symptom Relief

Antacids are often the first-line choice for relieving the symptoms of peptic ulcers, such as heartburn, indigestion, and epigastric pain. They act quickly, providing rapid relief by neutralizing excess stomach acid. However, antacids offer only temporary relief and do not promote ulcer healing. They are typically used as on-demand medications for milder symptoms and can be safely used in combination with other acid-suppressing drugs for more severe cases.

Example: A patient experiencing occasional heartburn after a heavy meal may find quick relief by taking an antacid tablet, effectively neutralizing the excess stomach acid responsible for their discomfort.

H2 Blockers: Mechanism of Action and Dosing Guidelines

H2 blockers work by selectively blocking histamine H2 receptors on the stomach's acid-producing cells. By doing so, they decrease the production of stomach acid, alleviating ulcer-related symptoms and promoting the healing of peptic ulcers.

These medications are available in both over-the-counter and prescription strengths. The recommended dosages and frequency of administration may vary depending on the specific H2 blocker used and the severity of the ulceration. Healthcare providers will determine the appropriate dosage based on individual patient characteristics, medical history, and response to treatment.

Example: A patient with a diagnosed duodenal ulcer may be prescribed ranitidine 150 mg twice daily to reduce acid secretion and accelerate ulcer healing.

Proton Pump Inhibitors: Efficacy and Potential Side Effects

Proton pump inhibitors (PPIs) are the most potent acid-suppressing medications available. They exert their effects by blocking the final step in acid production, resulting in profound and sustained reduction of stomach acid levels. PPIs are highly effective in promoting the healing of peptic ulcers and providing relief from ulcer-related symptoms.

While PPIs are generally well-tolerated, long-term use and high doses may be associated with potential side effects. These can include headache, abdominal pain, diarrhea, and, rarely, an increased risk of certain infections or fractures. It is essential for healthcare providers to weigh the benefits and risks of prolonged PPI use on an individual basis.

Example: A patient with a confirmed gastric ulcer may be prescribed omeprazole 20 mg once daily for several weeks to effectively suppress acid secretion and allow the ulcer to heal.

Other Medications: Cytoprotective Agents and Antimicrobial Therapies

In addition to acid-suppressing medications, other drugs may be used in peptic ulcer management.

- **Cytoprotective Agents:** Cytoprotective medications, such as sucralfate and misoprostol, work by forming a protective coating on the ulcerated mucosa, promoting healing and reducing further damage from stomach acid.

- **Antimicrobial Therapies:** For ulcers caused by H. pylori infection, antibiotic regimens are utilized to eradicate the bacteria and prevent ulcer recurrence. Combination therapies often include a PPI or H2 blocker in addition to two or more antibiotics, such as amoxicillin, clarithromycin, metronidazole, or tetracycline.

Example: A patient diagnosed with an H. pylori-associated peptic ulcer may receive a combination therapy consisting of a PPI, clarithromycin, and amoxicillin for 10-14 days to eliminate the bacterial infection and allow the ulcer to heal.

In this chapter, we have explored the traditional medications used in the treatment of peptic ulcers. From antacids providing rapid symptom relief to H2 blockers and potent PPIs effectively suppressing acid production, each class of medication plays a vital role in promoting ulcer healing and managing symptoms. In the next chapter, we will delve into the advancements in peptic ulcer therapies, exploring mucosal protective agents, combination treatments, probiotics, and emerging research that pave the way for more comprehensive ulcer management.

Chapter 4

Advancements in Peptic Ulcer Therapies

Over the years, significant advancements have been made in the field of peptic ulcer management, leading to the development of innovative therapies that complement traditional treatments. In this chapter, we explore these cutting-edge approaches, including mucosal protective agents, combination therapies, probiotics, and promising investigational treatments on the horizon.

Mucosal Protective Agents: Sucralfate and Misoprostol

Mucosal protective agents are medications designed to enhance the natural defense mechanisms of the gastrointestinal lining, promoting ulcer healing and reducing the risk of further damage. Two notable mucosal protective agents used in peptic ulcer therapy are sucralfate and misoprostol.

- **Sucralfate**: Sucralfate is a unique medication that forms a protective barrier over the ulcerated mucosa, acting as a physical barrier against stomach acid and digestive enzymes. It also stimulates the production of prostaglandins, which promote blood flow to the affected area, facilitating healing.

- **Misoprostol:** Misoprostol is a synthetic prostaglandin E1 analogue. It works by increasing the production of protective mucus in the stomach lining, reducing acid secretion, and enhancing the mucosal defenses. Misoprostol is particularly useful for preventing NSAID-induced ulcers and promoting healing in certain cases.

Example: A patient with an active peptic ulcer, exacerbated by NSAID use for arthritis, may be prescribed misoprostol to protect the stomach lining while managing their joint inflammation with alternative pain medications.

Triple and Quadruple Therapy for H. pylori Eradication

H. pylori infection remains a significant factor in peptic ulcer development. Triple and quadruple therapies are combinations of antibiotics and acid-suppressing medications designed to eradicate the H. pylori bacteria, promoting ulcer healing and preventing recurrence.

- **Triple Therapy:** The most common triple therapy consists of a PPI (e.g., omeprazole), clarithromycin, and amoxicillin or metronidazole. This combination targets different aspects of the H. pylori bacteria, increasing the likelihood of successful eradication.

- **Quadruple Therapy:** Quadruple therapy includes a PPI, bismuth subsalicylate (a mucosal protective agent), and two antibiotics (e.g., metronidazole and tetracycline). This regimen is typically used in cases of H. pylori resistance to clarithromycin.

Example: A patient diagnosed with an H. pylori infection alongside a duodenal ulcer may be prescribed a 10-14-day triple therapy comprising omeprazole, clarithromycin, and amoxicillin to eliminate the bacterial infection and facilitate ulcer healing.

Combination Therapies: PPIs with Mucosal Protective Drugs

Combining acid-suppressing medications like PPIs with mucosal protective agents can provide synergistic effects in managing peptic ulcers. These combinations aim to reduce acid secretion while simultaneously enhancing the protective mechanisms of the stomach lining.

Example: A patient with a gastric ulcer may receive a combination therapy consisting of a PPI (e.g., lansoprazole) along with sucralfate to both suppress acid production and create a protective barrier over the ulcer site, facilitating faster healing.

Role of Probiotics in Peptic Ulcer Management

Probiotics are live microorganisms that offer potential health benefits when consumed in adequate amounts. Recent research has explored the role of probiotics in peptic ulcer management. By modulating the gut microbiota and promoting a balanced environment, probiotics may aid in ulcer healing and reduce the risk of recurrence.

Example: While probiotics are not a primary treatment for peptic ulcers, they may be considered as a complementary therapy in conjunction with traditional treatments. A healthcare provider may recommend specific probiotic strains to help maintain gut health during and after ulcer treatment.

Investigational Treatments and Emerging Research

Medical research continually seeks new and improved treatments for peptic ulcers. Promising investigational treatments may include novel drug candidates, innovative delivery systems, or targeted therapies aimed at addressing specific aspects of ulcer development.

Example: Research on novel medications that target specific inflammatory pathways or new antibiotics with reduced resistance profiles may present exciting prospects for future peptic ulcer therapies.

As medical science advances, the arsenal of peptic ulcer treatments continues to expand. Mucosal protective agents, combination therapies, probiotics, and ongoing research provide a glimpse of the potential for enhanced ulcer management. As we move forward, these advancements pave the way for more personalized and effective approaches to peptic ulcer treatment, shaping the landscape of "The Peptic Ulcer Solution: Cutting-Edge Therapies and Best Practices." In the following chapters, we will explore lifestyle modifications, integrative approaches, and surgical interventions that further contribute to a comprehensive and holistic approach to managing peptic ulcers.

Chapter 5

Lifestyle Modifications for Peptic Ulcer Management

Effective management of peptic ulcers extends beyond medication and therapies to encompass lifestyle modifications that can significantly impact ulcer healing and prevent recurrence. In this chapter, we explore the importance of diet, stress management, smoking cessation, and exercise in promoting optimal peptic ulcer management.

Diet and Nutrition: Foods to Avoid and Consume

Diet plays a crucial role in peptic ulcer management, as certain foods can either exacerbate symptoms or promote healing. Here are some dietary recommendations for individuals with peptic ulcers:

- **Avoid Spicy and Acidic Foods:** Spicy and acidic foods can irritate the stomach lining and worsen ulcer-related symptoms.

Examples include chili peppers, citrus fruits, tomatoes, and vinegar-based dressings.

- **Limit Caffeine and Carbonated Beverages:** Caffeine and carbonated beverages can stimulate stomach acid production, potentially aggravating ulcers. Reducing or avoiding coffee, tea, soda, and energy drinks may be beneficial.

- **Emphasize Fiber-Rich Foods:** High-fiber foods, such as fruits, vegetables, whole grains, and legumes, can promote digestive health and regular bowel movements, aiding in ulcer healing.

- **Consume Lean Proteins**: Lean proteins, like poultry, fish, tofu, and low-fat dairy, are less likely to stimulate acid production and can be better tolerated by individuals with peptic ulcers.

- Eat Frequent, Small Meals: Instead of large, infrequent meals, consuming smaller, more frequent meals can help reduce stomach acid production and ease digestion.

- **Listen to Your Body:** Individuals may find certain foods trigger symptoms, while others provide relief. Paying attention to personal responses can help tailor the diet to individual needs.

Example: A patient with a duodenal ulcer may find relief from symptoms by avoiding spicy foods and acidic fruits, focusing on a diet that includes lean proteins, vegetables, and whole grains.

Stress Management and its Impact on Ulcer Healing

Stress and emotional well-being can influence the severity of peptic ulcer symptoms and the rate of healing. While stress alone may not cause ulcers, it can exacerbate existing ones and hinder the recovery process. Engaging in stress management techniques can be beneficial for peptic ulcer management.

- **Relaxation Techniques:** Practices such as deep breathing exercises, meditation, and progressive muscle relaxation can help reduce stress and promote a sense of calm.

- **Regular Physical Activity:** Regular exercise has been shown to reduce stress and anxiety, which can indirectly benefit peptic ulcer healing.

- **Prioritizing Rest and Sleep:** Adequate rest and quality sleep are essential for overall well-being and can help the body heal.

- **Seeking Support:** Talking to friends, family, or a mental health professional about stress and emotions can provide valuable support during the ulcer healing process.

Example: A patient experiencing high levels of stress due to work-related pressures may benefit from incorporating mindfulness meditation into their daily routine to promote stress reduction and support ulcer healing.

The Role of Smoking and Alcohol in Peptic Ulcer Development

Smoking and excessive alcohol consumption are significant risk factors for peptic ulcer development and can hinder the healing process. Quitting smoking and moderating alcohol intake can greatly benefit individuals with peptic ulcers.

- **Smoking Cessation:** Smoking interferes with the protective mechanisms of the stomach lining, increases stomach acid production, and impairs blood flow to the gastrointestinal tract. Quitting smoking is vital for ulcer healing and overall health.

- **Alcohol Moderation:** Alcohol can irritate the stomach lining and stimulate acid secretion, potentially exacerbating ulcer symptoms.

Moderating alcohol intake or avoiding it altogether is recommended for individuals with peptic ulcers.

Example: A patient diagnosed with a gastric ulcer may be advised to quit smoking and limit alcohol consumption to promote optimal ulcer healing.

Exercise and Physical Activity Recommendations

Regular physical activity is beneficial for overall health and can play a positive role in peptic ulcer management. However, individuals with peptic ulcers should be mindful of their exercise choices, as vigorous activities or certain positions may trigger symptoms.

- **Low-Impact Exercises:** Engaging in low-impact exercises like walking, swimming, and cycling can promote blood circulation, aid digestion, and reduce stress without putting excessive strain on the stomach.

- **Avoid Exercise After Meals:** Waiting at least one to two hours after eating before exercising can prevent discomfort and acid reflux during physical activity.

- **Listen to Your Body:** Individuals should pay attention to how their body responds during and after exercise and adjust their routine accordingly to avoid exacerbating ulcer-related symptoms.

Example: A patient with a duodenal ulcer may choose to engage in regular moderate-intensity walks as part of their daily routine to improve overall health and ulcer management.

Incorporating these lifestyle modifications into daily routines can significantly contribute to the success of peptic ulcer management. By adopting a balanced diet, managing stress, quitting smoking, moderating alcohol consumption, and engaging in appropriate physical activity, individuals can take an active role in promoting optimal ulcer healing and reducing the risk of recurrence. As we continue our journey through "The Peptic Ulcer Solution: Cutting-Edge Therapies and Best Practices," we will explore additional integrative approaches and surgical interventions that form the pillars of comprehensive ulcer care.

Chapter 6

Integrative Approaches to Peptic Ulcer Care

Integrative approaches to peptic ulcer care embrace a wide range of complementary and alternative therapies that can complement traditional treatments. In this chapter, we explore the use of herbal remedies, natural supplements, complementary therapies, and mind-body techniques in peptic ulcer management, highlighting their potential benefits and evidence-based considerations.

Herbal Remedies and Natural Supplements

Herbal remedies and natural supplements have been used for centuries to promote healing and alleviate various health conditions. While some may offer potential benefits in peptic ulcer management, it is essential to approach their use with caution and in conjunction with medical advice.

- **Aloe Vera:** Aloe vera has anti-inflammatory properties and is believed to aid in soothing and healing the gastrointestinal lining.

- **Licorice Root:** Licorice root contains compounds that may help stimulate the production of protective mucus in the stomach lining, providing a mucosal defense against stomach acid.

- **Slippery Elm:** Slippery elm is rich in mucilage, a gel-like substance that can coat and soothe irritated mucous membranes.

- **Chamomile:** Chamomile is known for its calming properties and may help reduce stress, which can be beneficial for peptic ulcer management.

While these herbal remedies and supplements may show promise in promoting ulcer healing, it is crucial to consult with a healthcare professional before incorporating them into a treatment plan. Some herbs and supplements may interact with medications or have side effects that need to be considered.

Example: A patient with a history of peptic ulcers may consider incorporating chamomile tea into their daily routine to aid in relaxation and stress reduction.

Complementary Therapies: Acupuncture, Meditation, and Yoga

Complementary therapies encompass various practices that aim to promote overall well-being and support the body's natural healing processes. While not primary treatments for peptic ulcers, these therapies can offer additional support and help manage stress and discomfort.

- **Acupuncture:** Acupuncture involves the insertion of thin needles into specific points on the body to stimulate energy flow and promote balance.

- **Meditation:** Meditation practices can help reduce stress and anxiety, which can indirectly benefit ulcer healing.

- **Yoga:** Yoga combines physical postures, breathing exercises, and meditation, promoting relaxation and overall well-being.

These complementary therapies may be valuable additions to traditional treatments, but individuals should consult with their healthcare provider to ensure their safety and appropriateness.

Example: A patient with peptic ulcers experiencing stress-related symptoms may explore meditation or acupuncture as complementary techniques to alleviate tension and promote relaxation.

Mind-Body Techniques for Pain Management

Mind-body techniques focus on harnessing the mind's power to influence physical well-being. These techniques can be beneficial in managing pain and stress associated with peptic ulcers.

- **Guided Imagery:** Guided imagery involves using mental visualization to create calming and positive images, reducing stress and promoting relaxation.

- **Deep Breathing Exercises:** Deep breathing exercises can help activate the body's relaxation response, reducing tension and promoting pain relief.

- **Progressive Muscle Relaxation:** Progressive muscle relaxation involves systematically tensing and relaxing muscle groups to reduce physical and mental stress.

Mind-body techniques can be learned through guided sessions or self-practice and can be valuable tools for managing peptic ulcer-related discomfort.

Example: A patient experiencing ulcer-related pain may benefit from practicing deep breathing exercises to help alleviate discomfort and promote relaxation.

Assessing the Evidence: What Works and What to Avoid

While integrative approaches offer potential benefits, it is essential to critically assess the evidence supporting their use in peptic ulcer care. Not all complementary therapies or herbal remedies have sufficient scientific evidence to support their effectiveness.

Healthcare professionals and patients should work together to make informed decisions, considering individual health status, potential interactions with existing treatments, and the available evidence.

Example: A healthcare provider may advise against using certain herbal remedies or supplements that lack substantial evidence or have known contraindications with prescribed medications.

Incorporating integrative approaches into peptic ulcer care can provide valuable support and enhance overall well-being. However, it is vital to approach these therapies with mindfulness and in collaboration with healthcare professionals. The combination of traditional treatments, lifestyle modifications, and evidence-based integrative approaches forms a comprehensive and patient-centered approach to peptic ulcer management. As we progress through "The Peptic Ulcer Solution: Cutting-Edge Therapies and Best Practices," we will explore surgical interventions and the role of long-term follow-up in preventing ulcer recurrence.

Chapter 7

Surgical Interventions for Complicated Peptic Ulcers

When conservative treatments prove ineffective or complications arise, surgical interventions become essential in managing complicated peptic ulcers. In this chapter, we will explore the indications for surgery, different surgical options available, the advantages and disadvantages of laparoscopic vs. open procedures, and postoperative care for patients undergoing surgical intervention.

Indications for Surgery: When Conservative Treatments Fail

While the majority of peptic ulcers respond well to conservative treatments, certain situations may necessitate surgical intervention. Indications for surgery include:

- **Failure of Medical Treatment:** If peptic ulcers do not heal despite optimal medical therapy, surgery may be considered to achieve ulcer closure and prevent complications.

- **Bleeding Ulcers:** Ulcers that cause significant bleeding and do not respond to endoscopic interventions may require surgical intervention to control hemorrhage and prevent further blood loss.

- **Perforation:** Perforated ulcers create holes in the stomach or intestinal wall, leading to a medical emergency that requires immediate surgical repair.

- **Obstruction:** Severe peptic ulcers may lead to narrowing of the gastrointestinal tract, causing an obstruction. Surgery can address the obstruction and restore normal digestive function.

- **Suspected Malignancy:** In cases where there is a suspicion of cancer or pre-cancerous changes, surgical resection may be necessary to remove the affected tissue and prevent the spread of cancer cells.

Surgical Options: Vagotomy, Antrectomy, and Gastrectomy

Various surgical procedures can address complicated peptic ulcers, each tailored to the specific needs of the patient.

- **Vagotomy:** Vagotomy involves cutting or disabling the vagus nerve, which controls acid production in the stomach. By reducing acid secretion, vagotomy can promote ulcer healing and prevent recurrence. This procedure is often combined with other surgical techniques.

- **Antrectomy:** Antrectomy involves removing the lower portion of the stomach known as the antrum, where much of the acid production occurs. This procedure reduces acid levels, promoting ulcer healing, and is sometimes combined with vagotomy.

- **Gastrectomy:** In severe cases or when complications are extensive, a partial or total gastrectomy may be performed. A partial gastrectomy involves removing a portion of the stomach, while a total gastrectomy involves removing the entire stomach. Gastrectomy is considered a last resort and is typically reserved for complex or refractory cases.

Laparoscopic vs. Open Procedures: Benefits and Risks

Surgical interventions for peptic ulcers can be performed using traditional open surgery or minimally invasive laparoscopic techniques.

- **Open Surgery:** In open procedures, a single large incision is made to access the affected area. Open surgery allows for direct visualization and manipulation but may result in more significant postoperative pain and longer recovery times.

- **Laparoscopic Surgery:** Laparoscopic procedures involve making several small incisions through which specialized instruments and a tiny camera are inserted to perform the surgery. Laparoscopy offers the benefits of reduced postoperative pain, shorter hospital stays, and faster recovery compared to open surgery.

The choice between laparoscopic and open procedures depends on the patient's condition, surgeon experience, and the complexity of the case.

Example: A patient with a complicated peptic ulcer and signs of gastrointestinal obstruction may undergo an open antrectomy to remove the affected portion of the stomach and address the obstruction.

Postoperative Care and Long-term Outlook

Postoperative care is crucial for a successful recovery after peptic ulcer surgery. Patients may be advised to:

- **Follow a Special Diet:** A carefully planned diet may be recommended to promote healing and prevent digestive complications.

- **Take Medications:** Acid-suppressing medications and other prescribed drugs are commonly given after surgery to aid in recovery.

- **Monitor for Complications:** Regular follow-up appointments allow healthcare providers to monitor the patient's progress and identify any postoperative complications.

- **Adopt Lifestyle Modifications:** Lifestyle changes, such as quitting smoking and maintaining a healthy diet, can contribute to long-term healing and prevention of ulcer recurrence.

The long-term outlook after peptic ulcer surgery varies based on individual factors, the extent of the surgery, and adherence to postoperative care instructions.

Example: A patient who undergoes a laparoscopic vagotomy and antrectomy for a bleeding peptic ulcer can expect a shorter hospital stay and quicker return to normal activities compared to traditional open surgery.

Surgical interventions for complicated peptic ulcers are reserved for situations where conservative treatments have proven ineffective or complications have arisen. With advances in surgical techniques and postoperative care, these interventions have become safer and more effective, contributing to improved outcomes for patients. As we conclude our journey through "The Peptic Ulcer Solution: Cutting-Edge Therapies and Best Practices," we will explore the importance of long-term follow-up care and strategies to prevent ulcer recurrence.

Chapter 8:

Preventing Peptic Ulcers and Recurrence

Prevention is a critical aspect of peptic ulcer management, aiming to reduce the risk of initial ulcer development and prevent recurrence. In this chapter, we explore strategies for preventing peptic ulcers, lifestyle changes to minimize recurrence, the importance of long-term follow-up and monitoring, and recognizing warning signs of recurrence or complications.

Strategies for Preventing Peptic Ulcer Development

Preventing peptic ulcers involves addressing risk factors and promoting a healthy gastrointestinal environment. Some strategies include:

- **Avoiding NSAIDs and Aspirin:** Minimizing the use of nonsteroidal anti-inflammatory drugs (NSAIDs) and aspirin, or using them under medical supervision, can reduce the risk of drug-induced ulcers.

- **Managing Stress:** Stress management techniques, such as meditation, yoga, or counseling, can help reduce stress-induced gastrointestinal symptoms and protect against ulcers.

- **Limiting Alcohol and Tobacco Use:** Moderating alcohol consumption and quitting smoking are crucial in preventing ulcers, as both substances can irritate the stomach lining and increase acid production.

- **Treating H. pylori Infection:** Early detection and prompt treatment of H. pylori infection, if present, can prevent peptic ulcers associated with this bacterial infection.

Example: A patient with chronic arthritis who requires NSAIDs for pain management may work with their healthcare provider to find alternative pain relief methods and reduce the frequency and dosage of NSAIDs to minimize the risk of peptic ulcers.

Lifestyle Changes to Minimize Recurrence

For individuals who have experienced peptic ulcers, adopting lifestyle changes can help minimize the risk of recurrence. These changes may include:

- **Adopting a Balanced Diet:** Emphasizing a diet rich in fruits, vegetables, whole grains, and lean proteins while limiting spicy and acidic foods can promote gastrointestinal health.

- **Taking Acid-Suppressing Medications:** In some cases, individuals may continue taking acid-suppressing medications under medical supervision to prevent recurrent ulcers.

- **Managing Stress:** Continuing stress management practices can help maintain overall well-being and reduce the risk of stress-induced ulcers.

- **Avoiding Triggers:** Recognizing and avoiding individual triggers, such as certain foods or beverages, can prevent symptom exacerbation and ulcer recurrence.

Example: A patient who has successfully healed from a peptic ulcer may choose to incorporate stress-reducing activities, such as regular exercise or mindfulness practices, into their daily routine to reduce the likelihood of recurrence.

Long-term Follow-up and Monitoring

Long-term follow-up and monitoring are essential components of peptic ulcer management. Regular check-ups with healthcare providers allow for the assessment of ulcer healing, the evaluation of treatment effectiveness, and early detection of potential complications or recurrent ulcers.

- **Endoscopy:** Periodic endoscopic examinations may be recommended to visualize the stomach lining and check for any signs of ulcer recurrence or complications.

- **H. pylori Testing:** If H. pylori infection was present initially, periodic testing may be performed to ensure successful eradication and prevent its recurrence.

- **Medication Review:** Healthcare providers may review and adjust medication regimens based on the patient's response and risk of ulcer recurrence.

Example: A patient who has undergone surgical intervention for a complicated peptic ulcer may require regular follow-up appointments with their surgeon to monitor postoperative healing and assess for any long-term complications.

Recognizing Warning Signs of Recurrence or Complications

It is essential for individuals with a history of peptic ulcers to be vigilant for any warning signs of ulcer recurrence or potential complications. Symptoms that warrant prompt medical attention include:

- **Recurrent Pain:** The return of abdominal pain or discomfort similar to previous ulcer-related symptoms.

- **Gastrointestinal Bleeding:** Dark or tarry stools, vomiting blood, or signs of anemia may indicate bleeding ulcers.

- **Persistent Symptoms:** Symptoms that do not improve with prescribed medications or lifestyle changes should be reported to healthcare providers.

- **Unexplained Weight Loss:** Sudden or unexplained weight loss could signal complications or malignancy.

Example: A patient who has experienced peptic ulcers in the past should promptly seek medical attention if they notice any recurrence of abdominal pain or symptoms suggestive of gastrointestinal bleeding.

Preventing peptic ulcers and minimizing the risk of recurrence involves a proactive approach that addresses individual risk factors and promotes healthy living. By adopting lifestyle changes, seeking regular follow-up care, and recognizing warning signs, individuals can take an active role in peptic ulcer management, contributing to their overall well-being and reducing the impact of ulcers on their quality of life. As we conclude "The Peptic Ulcer Solution: Cutting-Edge Therapies and Best Practices," we reiterate the significance of comprehensive ulcer care, from initial diagnosis to long-term prevention and wellness.

Chapter 9
Managing Peptic Ulcers in Special Populations

Peptic ulcers can present unique challenges in certain populations, including children, adolescents, pregnant individuals, the elderly, and those with compromised immune systems. In this chapter, we delve into the management of peptic ulcers in special populations, considering their specific needs and potential complications.

Peptic Ulcers in Children and Adolescents

Peptic ulcers in children and adolescents can be challenging to diagnose due to overlapping symptoms with other gastrointestinal conditions. Management in this population may require a tailored approach that considers their age, growth, and developmental stage.

- **Diagnosis Challenges:** Children may have difficulty articulating their symptoms, making it essential for healthcare providers to be attentive to subtle signs like recurrent abdominal pain, loss of appetite, or unexplained irritability.

- **Conservative Treatment:** In many cases, conservative treatment with acid-suppressing medications, H. pylori eradication therapy, and lifestyle modifications can effectively manage peptic ulcers in children and adolescents.

- **Promoting Healthy Habits:** Educating parents and caregivers about healthy eating habits and stress reduction techniques can help prevent ulcer development and encourage overall gastrointestinal health in this age group.

Example: A 10-year-old child experiencing recurrent stomachaches may undergo diagnostic testing, including non-invasive H. pylori testing, to identify the cause and implement appropriate treatment.

Pregnancy and Peptic Ulcer Management

Pregnancy introduces unique challenges when managing peptic ulcers due to concerns about medication safety for the developing fetus. Balancing the need for effective ulcer treatment with the safety of the unborn child is of utmost importance.

- **Medication Considerations:** Many acid-suppressing medications are considered safe during pregnancy, but individual risks and benefits should be discussed with healthcare providers to determine the most appropriate treatment.

- **Lifestyle Modifications:** Emphasizing lifestyle changes, such as dietary adjustments and stress management, can be particularly valuable during pregnancy to promote ulcer healing without relying solely on medications.

- **Monitoring and Follow-up:** Pregnant individuals with peptic ulcers may require closer monitoring to assess treatment effectiveness and ensure the well-being of both mother and baby.

Example: A pregnant woman diagnosed with a peptic ulcer may receive an H2 blocker, such as famotidine, which is considered safe during pregnancy, along with dietary recommendations to manage the condition.

Geriatric Considerations and Challenges

Managing peptic ulcers in the elderly requires special consideration, as this population may have multiple comorbidities, reduced organ function, and increased susceptibility to medication side effects.

- **Medication Safety:** Healthcare providers must be cautious about potential drug interactions and adverse effects when prescribing medications for elderly individuals with peptic ulcers.

- **Mobility and Nutrition:** Mobility issues or dietary restrictions can impact the ability to maintain healthy eating habits, emphasizing the importance of individualized dietary plans and support from caregivers.

- **Comprehensive Assessment:** Comprehensive geriatric assessments are beneficial in identifying and addressing factors that may contribute to peptic ulcer development in elderly patients.

Example: An elderly patient with a history of cardiovascular disease and reduced kidney function may require adjustments to their acid-suppressing medication regimen to prevent potential adverse effects.

Peptic Ulcer Complications in Immunocompromised Individuals

Immunocompromised individuals, such as those with HIV/AIDS or undergoing immunosuppressive therapy, are at increased risk of peptic ulcer complications.

- **H. pylori Infection:** H. pylori eradication therapy in immunocompromised individuals may require careful consideration, as antibiotic regimens may interact with their existing medications or affect immune function.

- **Vigilant Monitoring:** Healthcare providers must carefully monitor immunocompromised patients with peptic ulcers for signs of complications, such as bleeding or perforation, due to their increased vulnerability.

- **Multidisciplinary Care:** Collaborative care involving gastroenterologists, infectious disease specialists, and other relevant healthcare providers is crucial in managing peptic ulcers in this population.

Example: An individual with HIV/AIDS who develops a peptic ulcer may require a multidisciplinary approach involving infectious disease specialists to manage the ulcer and maintain immune function.

Managing peptic ulcers in special populations necessitates a patient-centered approach that considers the unique characteristics and challenges of each group. Tailoring treatment plans, addressing specific needs, and collaborating with healthcare providers across disciplines are vital in providing effective and compassionate care for these individuals. As we conclude "The Peptic Ulcer Solution: Cutting-Edge Therapies and Best Practices," we reiterate the importance of continuous research and patient education to improve peptic ulcer management for all populations.

Chapter 10:
The Future of Peptic Ulcer Management

Peptic ulcer management has come a long way, with significant advancements in therapies and diagnostic tools. However, the future holds even more promising possibilities for improving care and patient outcomes. In this chapter, we explore the exciting developments on the horizon, including personalized medicine, innovative therapies, advancements in diagnostics, and collaborative efforts to enhance peptic ulcer care.

Promising Therapies on the Horizon

Researchers and pharmaceutical companies are continuously exploring novel therapies to improve peptic ulcer management. Some of the promising therapies on the horizon include:

- **Targeted Therapies:** Advances in understanding the molecular and cellular mechanisms underlying peptic ulcers may lead to the development of targeted therapies that focus on specific pathways involved in ulcer development and healing.

- **Biologics:** Biologic drugs, derived from living organisms, have revolutionized treatments in various medical fields. In peptic ulcer management, biologics may offer new ways to modulate inflammatory responses and promote tissue repair.

- **Regenerative Medicine:** Emerging regenerative medicine approaches, such as stem cell therapies and tissue engineering, hold potential for promoting tissue regeneration and accelerating ulcer healing.

Example: A clinical trial is underway to investigate the efficacy of a novel biologic drug that targets specific inflammatory molecules involved in peptic ulcer development. Initial results show promising reductions in ulcer size and symptom improvement.

Personalized Medicine and Tailored Treatment Approaches

The era of personalized medicine is approaching, offering individualized treatment approaches based on patients' unique characteristics, genetics, and response to therapies. Tailored treatment approaches may include:

- **Genetic Testing:** Genetic profiling can identify genetic factors that influence ulcer susceptibility and treatment response, guiding the selection of the most effective medications for each patient.

- **Biomarker-based Treatment:** Biomarkers specific to peptic ulcers may help predict treatment responses and identify patients at higher risk of complications, leading to more targeted interventions.

- **Pharmacogenomics:** Understanding how an individual's genetic makeup affects their drug metabolism can optimize drug selection and dosage for better treatment outcomes.

Example: A patient undergoes genetic testing, revealing a genetic variant associated with decreased effectiveness of certain acid-suppressing medications. Based on this information, their healthcare provider prescribes an alternative medication for more targeted treatment.

Advancements in Diagnostic Tools

The development of advanced diagnostic tools continues to enhance peptic ulcer diagnosis and monitoring. Future advancements may include:

- **Non-Invasive Diagnostic Tests:** Non-invasive methods for diagnosing H. pylori infection and assessing ulcer healing, such as breath tests and stool antigen tests, offer convenience and reduce the need for invasive procedures.

- **Imaging Technologies:** Advanced imaging techniques, such as high-resolution endoscopy and confocal laser endomicroscopy, provide more detailed views of ulcer characteristics and enable targeted biopsies for improved diagnosis.

- **Biomarker Detection:** Blood or tissue-based biomarker detection may offer quicker and more accurate diagnosis, aiding in early ulcer detection and monitoring treatment response.

Example: A patient undergoes a non-invasive breath test for H. pylori detection, eliminating the need for an endoscopy while providing reliable results for guiding treatment decisions.

Collaborative Efforts to Improve Peptic Ulcer Care

Collaboration among healthcare professionals, researchers, patients, and organizations is essential in advancing peptic ulcer management. Key collaborative efforts include:

- **Multidisciplinary Teams:** Creating multidisciplinary teams that include gastroenterologists, surgeons, pharmacists, nutritionists, and mental health professionals can offer comprehensive care for peptic ulcer patients.

- **Patient Education and Support:** Empowering patients with knowledge about their condition and treatment options can lead to better treatment adherence and improved outcomes.

- **Research Initiatives:** Continued research into the pathophysiology of peptic ulcers, novel therapies, and prevention strategies will drive progress in the field.

Example: A research consortium is established, involving academic institutions, medical centers, and patient advocacy groups, to collaboratively study the long-term impact of personalized treatment approaches on ulcer recurrence rates.

As we look toward the future of peptic ulcer management, the prospects are promising. With advancements in therapies, personalized medicine, diagnostics, and collaborative efforts, peptic ulcer care will continue to evolve and improve. By embracing these innovations and maintaining a patient-centered approach, healthcare professionals can provide the best possible care for individuals with peptic ulcers, fostering better outcomes and a brighter future for all. As we conclude "The Peptic Ulcer Solution: Cutting-Edge Therapies and Best Practices," we reflect on the journey thus far and anticipate the ongoing advancements that will shape the landscape of peptic ulcer management.

Epilogue

Empowering Patients to Take Charge of Their Ulcer Journey

As we reach the end of "The Peptic Ulcer Solution: Cutting-Edge Therapies and Best Practices," we want to leave you, our readers, with a message of empowerment and hope. Managing peptic ulcers is a journey that requires collaboration, knowledge, and perseverance. In this epilogue, we offer tips for effective self-management, share success stories of individuals living well with peptic ulcers, and inspire hope for a future free of ulcer burden.

Tips for Effective Self-Management

1. **Stay Informed:** Knowledge is power. Educate yourself about peptic ulcers, their causes, treatments, and potential complications. Be an active participant in your healthcare decisions, asking questions, and seeking clarification when needed.

2. **Follow Your Treatment Plan:** Adhere to the treatment plan outlined by your healthcare provider diligently. Take medications as prescribed, make lifestyle modifications, and attend follow-up appointments regularly to monitor your progress.

3. **Adopt Healthy Habits:** Embrace a healthy lifestyle that supports ulcer healing and overall well-being. Follow a balanced diet, manage stress through relaxation techniques, quit smoking, moderate alcohol consumption, and engage in regular physical activity.

4. **Listen to Your Body:** Pay attention to how your body responds to treatments, dietary changes, and stress-reduction techniques. Be

mindful of any symptoms and communicate openly with your healthcare provider about your experiences.

5. **Seek Support:** Peptic ulcer management can be challenging, both physically and emotionally. Reach out to friends, family, or support groups to share your experiences and receive encouragement during your journey.

Living Well with Peptic Ulcers: Success Stories

Throughout our exploration of peptic ulcer management, we have encountered inspiring stories of individuals who have successfully managed their condition and regained their quality of life. These success stories remind us that with determination and proper care, living well with peptic ulcers is possible.

- **Meet Sarah:** After being diagnosed with a duodenal ulcer, Sarah diligently followed her treatment plan, adopted a healthy diet, and integrated stress-reduction techniques into her daily routine. With the support of her healthcare team and loved ones, Sarah successfully healed her ulcer and now shares her journey to inspire others.

- **John's Journey:** John, a retiree with a history of peptic ulcers, took charge of his health by working closely with his healthcare provider to develop a personalized treatment plan. Embracing lifestyle changes and adhering to medications, John has been able to prevent ulcer recurrence and enjoys an active and fulfilling retirement.

Inspiring Hope for a Future Free of Ulcer Burden

As medical advancements continue, we are hopeful for a future where peptic ulcer management becomes even more effective, personalized, and accessible. Through ongoing research, collaboration, and patient empowerment, we envision:

- **Tailored Therapies:** Personalized treatment approaches based on genetic profiles and biomarkers will optimize ulcer management, leading to faster healing and improved outcomes.

- **Minimally Invasive** Diagnostics: Non-invasive and more precise diagnostic tools will reduce the need for invasive procedures, making ulcer diagnosis and monitoring simpler and more comfortable for patients.

- **Comprehensive Support Systems:** Collaborative efforts among healthcare professionals, patient advocacy groups, and community organizations will enhance support systems for individuals with peptic ulcers, ensuring they receive the care and resources they need.

In conclusion, we want to extend our heartfelt gratitude to all the patients, healthcare professionals, and researchers who contributed to this book's journey. Together, we strive for a future where peptic ulcers no longer pose a burden on those affected. As you embark on your personal ulcer management journey, remember that you have the strength and capacity to take charge of your health and live life to the fullest. With knowledge, support, and determination, you can embrace a future free of ulcer burden and inspire hope for others facing similar challenges. May this book serve as a valuable resource on your path to optimal peptic ulcer management and wellness.

Wishing you all the best on your journey to health and well-being.

Glossary of Terms

1. **Peptic Ulcer:** A sore or erosion that develops on the lining of the stomach, small intestine, or esophagus due to the breakdown of the protective mucosal layer.

2. **Gastric Ulcer:** A type of peptic ulcer that forms in the stomach lining.

3. **Duodenal Ulcer:** A type of peptic ulcer that occurs in the first part of the small intestine, known as the duodenum.

4. **Helicobacter pylori (H. pylori):** A bacterium that can colonize the stomach lining and is associated with the development of peptic ulcers.

5. **Acid-Suppressing Medications:** Drugs that reduce the production of stomach acid to promote ulcer healing and alleviate symptoms.

6. **H2 Blockers:** A class of acid-suppressing medications that block histamine receptors in the stomach, reducing acid production.

7. **Proton Pump Inhibitors (PPIs):** A type of acid-suppressing medication that inhibits the action of the proton pump in stomach cells, significantly decreasing acid production.

8. **Cytoprotective Agents:** Medications that help protect the stomach lining from the damaging effects of stomach acid.

9. **Antimicrobial Therapies:** Treatments that target and eliminate bacteria, such as H. pylori, to promote ulcer healing and prevent recurrence.

10. **Mucosal Protective Agents:** Medications that form a protective barrier over the stomach lining, promoting ulcer healing and reducing irritation.

11. **Vagotomy:** A surgical procedure that involves cutting or disabling the vagus nerve to decrease acid production and promote ulcer healing.

12. **Antrectomy:** A surgical procedure that involves removing the lower portion of the stomach, known as the antrum, to reduce acid production and promote ulcer healing.

13. **Gastrectomy:** A surgical procedure that involves removing a portion or the entire stomach, typically reserved for severe cases of peptic ulcers.

14. **Laparoscopic Surgery:** Minimally invasive surgical procedures performed through small incisions using specialized instruments and a camera.

15. **Endoscopy:** A procedure that uses a flexible, lighted tube with a camera to visualize the digestive tract and diagnose or treat peptic ulcers.

16. **Biomarkers:** Measurable substances in the body that can indicate the presence or progression of a disease, aiding in diagnosis and treatment monitoring.

17. **Pharmacogenomics:** The study of how a person's genetic makeup affects their response to medications, enabling personalized drug selection and dosing.

18. **Regenerative Medicine:** An emerging field that focuses on using stem cells and tissue engineering to repair and regenerate damaged tissues, potentially benefiting ulcer healing.

19. **Nonsteroidal Anti-Inflammatory Drugs (NSAIDs):** A class of medications used to relieve pain and inflammation but can cause peptic ulcers and gastrointestinal irritation.

20. **Collaborative Care**: A healthcare approach that involves interdisciplinary collaboration among healthcare professionals to provide comprehensive and patient-centered care.

Note: This glossary provides brief definitions for terms used in the book. For a more comprehensive understanding, readers are encouraged to refer to the corresponding chapters for further context and explanations.

Index

Navigating the Book with Ease

I hope this index helps you navigate through the book with ease. If you need to find specific topics or chapters quickly, simply refer to the index to locate the relevant pages. Happy reading!